1,000 Things to Do with your Child

A Checklist for Strange Parents

To Valentina and Emma,

'Willing to throw your children out the window is fair. Throwing them out is not.'

José Pedro Lorca

Introduction to the book

Welcome

Dear parents,

Thanks for purchasing this book. I hope you enjoy it. If you have friends to share this work with, do it and I will be grateful for the rest of my life. Just kidding. I couldn't care less. I have got a job and other sources of income. Theft, for example.

Now, since you have kids your time is priceless. So, don't waste any and let's jump straight to it.

Disclaimers

Here I need to make some important disclaimers for all readers.

This book doesn't define you as a parent. It is not about being a good mom or dad. Even if you achieved checking all the activities of this book, that wouldn't define you as a parent. I have always been a quality over quantity supporter and this checklist is just a game. Never forget this.

Obviously, if you barely check off 15% of all the things that are listed here, you should consider leaving your child to the authorities to be raised by someone else. You really suck. Just kidding. It's normal to suck if you have kids. Just kidding, again.

Anyway, even in the case you strongly commit yourself to this checklist, don't take this book too seriously. I strongly recommend not going crazy on every single activity. Just check them and if they don't fit you, or if it's too late to do them, just let them go as something you simply didn't do. Again, this book is just a tool to look back and forward and see your life from a different point of view. Mine. So, really, don't take it seriously.

The book includes some of the most common things for each stage of growth of any normal kid. And when I say 'normal' it means 'normal'. Don't get angry if your child can't run or climb a tree: it's not my fault. You can still try out everything with some creative distinctions. It will be great anyway.

While reading this book, you could suddenly feel the urge to throw it away. Please, in case you do so, use the paper bin unless you're reading on an E-reader. Some of the readers might also feel the urge to add something personal to my checklist. That's why a good 20% of the total amount of activities (that is 200 activities) is left to you. 200 activities in 15 years. It's about one activity per month. If you don't die or disappear, you could do that.

In the next paragraphs I will explain how to use this book.

How to use this book

In this book you will find a list of activities that you could do with your child (or children) from the early stages to their adolescence. In brief, from 0 to 15 years old. Now you have a reason to survive another 15 years. That's worth the money you paid for the book.

First of all, you need a pencil. Don't use a pen, it's against the rules. I'm joking. Instead, I recommend to check the activities with colorful markers. The book will look nicer. If you are reading on an E-book, find an electronic way to check the list.

The book is structured in 7 chapters and every chapter has got a brief introduction because you didn't just buy a checklist. This one is a proper book!

Anyway, there are 1,000 (one thousand!) activities that follow the life of your child from 0 to 15 years old and give you suggestions for interesting things to do.

The book is quite intuitive to use. If you have done the activity, check it. And that is all.

In the next paragraphs I will focus on the virtues of this book.

The virtues of this book

What is a checklist? It's a list of things you need to check. Fine, now, why should we need a checklist? Because we tend to forget. Moreover, we tend to pretend we forget. In a word, we procrastinate.

So, the checklist will give you the opportunity to kill the procrastinator that lives in you. Plus, you will also remember everything you did for your children. To throw it back to their face when they are grown up.

Too often we forget to focus on how many things we do. So, these are some of the virtues of this book.

1. It is a checklist for the things that you could do with your kids in the future. If they feel bored on a rainy afternoon, just take the book and find one of the activities that I suggest.
2. It can be used as a checklist for the things that you have already done. So, check them all. No problem if your kid is 4, 7 or 12 years old. You still have lots of interesting suggestions to implement. And, of course, you can always go back and check what's missing.
3. It gives a bunch of ideas for new activities to do. Have I already said that?

4. It is a sort of family portrait for the things that you did with your family, just like a photo album. In a few years you will look back and see how much time you spent with your family before everything spoilt. It will be a moment of sweet sadness, I promise.
5. It is a time and stage reminder. Being a parent is a long run. So, don't take it fast and enjoy the ride. This checklist will show you what to expect and what not to expect at every single stage of your child's life.
6. It becomes a personal memory. You can track all the activities that I endorse, and you can add more details, such as a date or a specific memory that you have. It will turn this book into a diary. Moreover, I decided to leave some space for you to fill at the end of some chapters. This book can be read in a few hours, but it is thought out to be finished in years. So don't be hasty.

And finally,

7. I live in Rome, Italy, and I strongly recommend you to come and visit. At the end of the book you will find a list of 50 activities to do in the Eternal City with your family.

Fine, I think we can start! You now know everything you need to explore this book and enjoy the checklist as you like!

I hope you really experience this checklist the best you can. Good luck and I'll see you at the end of the book!

Chapter One

0 – 1 years old

At the same time, this is the best and the worst period of your life as a parent. Your child is just a baby. He or she doesn't move much but everything around you goes really fast. Your life is now full of worries, stress and intrusive relatives. It is the best period to check the things that happen, because it's the period when you are probably doing and forgetting most. And kids can't remember on their own at this stage of life.

1. ☐ Carry out the delivery or witness it.
2. ☐ Witness the first washing after birth.
3. ☐ Receive the hug of the relatives.
4. ☐ Introduce the baby to the grandparents.

5. ☐ Introduce the baby to uncles, aunts and cousins.

6. ☐ Spend the first night with your baby.

7. ☐ Worry or don't worry if the baby grows enough.

8. ☐ Wet the baby's head with a round of drinks.

9. ☐ Witness the fall of the umbilical cord.

10. ☐ Take the first stroll with the pram.

11. ☐ Show the baby his/her new home.

12. ☐ Talk *with* the baby, not *to* the baby.

13. ☐ Call the baby by his/her name.

14. ☐ Say 'please' and 'thanks' to the baby.

15. ☐ Change the baby's diaper.

16. ☐ Give the baby his/her first bath.

17. ☐ Comfort the baby when he/she cries.

18. ☐ Give the baby a massage.

19. ☐ Rock the baby in your arms.

20. ☐ Carry the baby on your back.

21. ☐ Cut the baby's hair.

22. ☐ Cut the baby's nails.

23. ☐ Nurse the baby with a bottle.

24. ☐ Scratch the baby.

25. ☐ Write a diary for the most relevant moments.

26. ☐ Introduce him/her to other babies.

27. ☐ Comb the baby's hair.

28. ☐ Teach the baby to walk.

29. ☐ Teach the baby to say 'hello' and 'goodbye'.

30. ☐ Teach the baby to say 'please' and 'thank you'.

31. ☐ Witness the first time the baby calls you.

32. ☐ Comfort the baby when he/she cries at night.

33. ☐ Teach the baby to climb steps.

34. ☐ Feed the ducks in a pond.

35. ☐ Make soap bubbles.

36. ☐ Play with your hands and the baby's face (nose, mouth, ears and so on).

37. ☐ Watch some TV together.

38. ☐ Make a video call with your baby.

39. ☐ Let your baby try lemon juice.

40. ☐ Cook for your baby.

41. ☐ Let your baby listen to classical music, from Mozart to Morricone.

42. ☐ Visit great-grandparents, wherever they are.

43. ☐ Cuddle your baby with your partner.

44. ☐ Take your baby to meet Santa Claus.

45. ☐ Teach the baby to count.

46. ☐ Take pictures of your baby and keep them for you.

47. ☐ Take picture with friends and relatives.

48. ☐ Make the baby burp.

49. ☐ Get your baby to fart.

50. ☐ Clean the baby's nose.

51. ☐ Get some vomit on your clothes.

52. ☐ Make effort to dodge baby's pee.

53. ☐ Make the baby's first video on camera.

54. ☐ See the first smiles.

55. ☐ Rinse the nose with that big syringe of solution.

56. ☐ Suck snot with a small pump.

57. ☐ Breastfeed.

58. ☐ Feed the mum while she is breastfeeding.

59. ☐ Let your child suck your finger to calm down.

60. ☐ Follow the pulse of blood from the 'fontanel'.

61. ☐ Put a speaker on the baby's belly and let it play music.
62. ☐ Tell stories.
63. ☐ Kiss the baby.
64. ☐ Clean the baby with cold water.
65. ☐ Swing the baby.
66. ☐ Carry the pram up and down the stairs.
67. ☐ Pee while holding the baby.
68. ☐ Hear the baby's first sounds.
69. ☐ Sing songs to the baby.
70. ☐ Feel proud.
71. ☐ Praise the baby before strangers.
72. ☐ Have sex with your partner while the baby is sleeping.
73. ☐ Let your baby listen to the radio, to podcast and TV shows.

74. ☐ Head butt the wall when the baby doesn't sleep.
75. ☐ Celebrate your first Father's Day or Mother's Day.
76. ☐ Celebrate your first birthday as a parent.
77. ☐ Keep the baby still during the vaccine.
78. ☐ Give him/her some baby food.
79. ☐ Tear paper to let the baby hear the sound.
80. ☐ Take an elevator with the baby.
81. ☐ Take a bus with the baby.
82. ☐ Take a train with the baby.
83. ☐ Take a plane with the baby.
84. ☐ Enter a church with the baby.
85. ☐ Enter a synagogue with a baby.
86. ☐ Enter a mosque with a baby.
87. ☐ Witness the appearing of the first tooth.
88. ☐ Bring the baby to the swimming pool.

89. ☐ Bring the baby to the sea.

90. ☐ Anesthetize the baby while feeding him/her.

91. ☐ Read a newspaper while the baby is sleeping.

92. ☐ Play him/her some music instrument.

93. ☐ Bring your baby to your workplace.

94. ☐ Witness the first time the baby sits without leaning on his/her hands.

95. ☐ Witness the first time the baby understands a "No".

96. ☐ Witness some letters: B. P. K.

97. ☐ Bring the baby to the nursery school.

98. ☐ Let the baby hurt you.

99. ☐ Put the baby in a rucksack and go low altitude trekking with your partner.

100. ☐ Dry the baby's hair.

101. ☐ Let the baby blow raspberries in your face while feeding him/her.
102. ☐ Teach the baby the "up" position and the "down" position.
103. ☐ Witness the baby laughing.
104. ☐ Witness the baby complaining.
105. ☐ Teach the baby to put objects in the correct position.
106. ☐ Let the baby press buttons on the elevator.
107. ☐ Show you are calm when the baby cries or gets hurt.
108. ☐ Let the baby bite you.
109. ☐ Push the baby on the swing.
110. ☐ Have a shower together with the baby.
111. ☐ Put the baby in the closet for few seconds.
112. ☐ Play with stickers.
113. ☐ Play with dolls.

114. ☐ Read the baby some cardboard books.

115. ☐ Create some rituals with your baby.

116. ☐ Save your baby's life at least once.

117. ☐ Remove plastic from your baby's mouth.

118. ☐ Make videos of your baby and keep them.

119. ☐ Teach the baby to blow candles and hot food.

120. ☐ Witness the baby's first steps.

121. ☐ Hear the baby's voice.

122. ☐ Get the baby's first kiss.

123. ☐ Give your baby a high five.

124. ☐ Hear the baby's first words.

125. ☐ Let the baby play some notes on a piano.

126. ☐ Get your baby's hand and foot prints.

127. ☐ Walk out alone with your baby.

128. ☐ Teach the baby some animal sounds.

129. ☐ Witness your baby saying hello to the people.
130. ☐ Witness your baby taking some spoons of food without any help.
131. ☐ Let the baby smell things like flowers or feet.
132. ☐ Play with flashcards.
133. ☐ Put your baby on a baby seat and go for a ride on a bike.
134. ☐ Break Easter eggs together.
135. ☐ Empty the washing machine together.
136. ☐ Hang clothes together.
137. ☐ Wean your baby off his/her pacifier.
138. ☐ Buy a doll or a puppet for your baby.
139. ☐ Have a jog with your baby in the stroller.
140. ☐ Teach the baby to say how old is he/she.

141. ☐ Teach the baby to use the toilet bowl as adults do.

142. ☐ Play with ice.

143. ☐ Go for a ride on a carousel.

144. ☐ Put the baby inside irrigators gush in a park.

145. ☐ Teach the baby some Spanish words.

146. ☐ Witness your baby sitting and eating on regular chairs.

147. ☐ Let your baby go on a slide.

148. ☐ Witness your baby climbing the slide.

149. ☐ Witness your baby telling someone his/her name.

150. ☐ Let your baby climb a rope net.

Now, some space for you to fill…

151. ☐ _____

152. ☐ _____

153. ☐ _____

154. ☐ _____

155. ☐ _____

156. ☐ _____

157. ☐ _____

158. ☐ _____

159. ☐ _____

160. ☐ _____

161. ☐ _____

162. ☐ _____

163. ☐ _____

164. ☐ _____

165. ☐ _____

166. ☐ _____

167. ☐ _____

168. ☐ _____

169. ☐ _____

170. ☐ _____

171. ☐ _____

172. ☐ _____

173. ☐ _____

174. ☐ _____

175. ☐ _____

176. ☐ _____

177. ☐ _____

178. ☐ _____

179. ☐ _____

180. ☐ _____

181. ☐ _____

182. ☐ _____

183. ☐ _____

184. ☐ _____

185. ☐ _____

186. ☐ _____

187. ☐ _____

188. ☐ _____

189. ☐ _____

190. ☐ _____

191. ☐ _____

192. ☐ _____

193. ☐ _____

194. ☐ _____

195. ☐ _____

196. ☐ _____

197. ☐ _____

198. ☐ _____

199. ☐ _____

200. ☐ _____

Chapter Two

2 – 5 years old

By this time, your child is no longer a baby. Children at this stage clearly express personal wishes and tend to be quite self-centred. So, you need to involve yourself even more if you want to keep pace. Don't get confused. You can still manipulate them as you like. Anyway, I suggest three principles: one, when you play with them, let them decide; two, anytime you can negotiate, do it; three, when there shouldn't be any discussion at all, just be authoritative and do your job.

201.   ☐ Blow out the candles for the second birthday.

202.   ☐ Toilet train your child.

203. ☐ Wean them off their pacifier.

204. ☐ Stimulate your child to differentiate colours.

205. ☐ Show your child if an object floats or sinks.

206. ☐ Start introducing some abstract concepts.

207. ☐ Make a tower with blocks.

208. ☐ Let your child hear your heartbeat with his/her head on your chest.

209. ☐ Teach numbers and count things with your child.

210. ☐ Show pride for the important goals that your child has reached so far.

211. ☐ Let your child make a portrait of you.

212. ☐ Paint a stone with your child.

213. ☐ Tell bedtime stories.

214. ☐ Write a song and sing it to your child.

215. ☐ Eat pizza in a restaurant.

216. ☐ Teach the child the National Anthem.

217. ☐ Let your child give some coins to street artists if he/she likes their work.
218. ☐ Teach the child some prayers and gratitude in general.
219. ☐ Teach the child the importance of space organization and order.
220. ☐ Teach the child good manners and how to detect bad manners around.
221. ☐ Read the child some Roald Dahl's books.
222. ☐ Educate the child to the respect the environment and how to recycle.
223. ☐ Give the child a book with pictures.
224. ☐ Let the child help you in a market when you buy food.
225. ☐ Tickle your child.
226. ☐ Eat an ice-cream without getting dirty.
227. ☐ Bring your child to a big toy shop.

228. ☐ Bring your child to an amusement park.

229. ☐ Play fight on the bed.

230. ☐ Invent a special greeting to share with your child.

231. ☐ Show your child how to applaud and show appreciation.

232. ☐ Teach the child how to whistle.

233. ☐ Teach the child how to gargle.

234. ☐ Take a tram with your kid.

235. ☐ Teach the child how to cross the street.

236. ☐ Teach the child how to kick a ball with both feet.

237. ☐ Give the child a wallet to keep money.

238. ☐ Teach your child how to write his/her name

239. ☐ Teach your child how to tie laces.

240. ☐ Read the newspaper while your child is playing alone.

241. ☐ Teach your child to read some letters.
242. ☐ Teach your child to get dressed on his/her own.
243. ☐ Teach your child the position of left and right.
244. ☐ Teach your child to ride a bike.
245. ☐ Teach your child to go on skates.
246. ☐ Teach your child to go on a push scooter.
247. ☐ Give your child a recorder and let him/her play.
248. ☐ Teach your child how to pet a cat.
249. ☐ Teach your child to fold clothes.
250. ☐ Teach your child how to drink from a drinking fountain.
251. ☐ Watch cartoons together.
252. ☐ Watch animation films together.
253. ☐ Watch documentaries together.

254. ☐ Watch a sport match together on TV.

255. ☐ Go to a zoo with the kid.

256. ☐ Go to a vegetable garden with your child.

257. ☐ Plant some seeds at home.

258. ☐ Decorate a Christmas tree, or any other religious ritual for winter time.

259. ☐ Make a brother or sister for your child.

260. ☐ Let your child smell beer, wine and whiskey. Just smell.

261. ☐ Make a costume for carnival.

262. ☐ Collect all kind of personal and important objects and show them to your child.

263. ☐ Show your child some old pictures of yours.

264. ☐ Teach your child the importance of reading.

265. ☐ Tell your child about the time you fell in love with your partner.

266. ☐ Teach your child the alphabet.

267. ☐ Make some science experiments.
268. ☐ Play a memory game with your kid.
269. ☐ Make some temporary tattoos.
270. ☐ Teach him/her all the road signs.
271. ☐ Discover together all the things your child can do while you can't anymore.
272. ☐ Play with a ball.
273. ☐ Bring your child to see fireworks.
274. ☐ Play with dice.
275. ☐ Play with coins.
276. ☐ Play hide and seek.
277. ☐ Encourage your child to participate in some kind of sport (swimming, dance, basketball...)
278. ☐ Write on a surface with pavement chalk.
279. ☐ Dig a huge hole in the sand.
280. ☐ Make a snowman.
281. ☐ Play bingo together.

282. ☐ Bring the child to the racecourse.

283. ☐ Bring your child to the circus.

284. ☐ Watch the clouds with your child.

285. ☐ On the beach, make a sand castle.

286. ☐ Measure his/her height on a wall.

287. ☐ Teach your child some group dance.

288. ☐ Pretend you are a professional diver and have a competition in a swimming pool.

289. ☐ Visit some friends who live far from home.

290. ☐ Do some easy mountain trekking together.

291. ☐ Start telling jokes.

292. ☐ Start telling easy riddles.

293. ☐ Teach some new Spanish words.

294. ☐ Eat almonds and all kind of nuts.

295. ☐ Let your child dust his/her bedroom.

296. ☐ Let your child water the plants.

297. ☐ Make a race track on the floor with some tape.
298. ☐ go around the house with your eyes closed.
299. ☐ Smell all kinds of food.
300. ☐ Hide an object in the room and ask your child to search for it.
301. ☐ See the sky at night with your child.
302. ☐ Let your child pour liquids from one place to another.
303. ☐ Let your child tighten bolt with his/her hands.
304. ☐ *Amar es Combatir*, by Manà. Let him/her listen to it.
305. ☐ Play the drums with kitchen pots.
306. ☐ Let your child step on you.
307. ☐ Teach your child how to stay seated while dining.

308. ☐ Go with your child to a birthday party.

309. ☐ Get dressed for Halloween.

310. ☐ Start teaching how to play chess.

311. ☐ Draw the family tree.

312. ☐ Make paper planes.

313. ☐ Leave your child for one night at his/her grandparents' house.

314. ☐ Make some origami animals.

315. ☐ Bring your child to an aquarium.

316. ☐ Play with paper and glue.

317. ☐ Let your child jump on trampolines.

318. ☐ Organise a treasure hunt for your child and his/her friends.

319. ☐ Go to a theatre play for children.

320. ☐ Go camping with the family.

321. ☐ Let your child ride a pony.

322. ☐ Write a picture book with your child using photos and drawings.
323. ☐ Make a drawing with watercolours.
324. ☐ Climb a tree.
325. ☐ Teach the basic opposites (tall/short, fast/slow...and so on).
326. ☐ Have dinner with another family.
327. ☐ Take a funicular railway.
328. ☐ Show your child how to stay balanced on one leg.
329. ☐ Climb a tower together.
330. ☐ Watch a magic show.
331. ☐ Bring your child to the car wash.
332. ☐ Make birthday cards for new friends.
333. ☐ Leave your child with a babysitter and go out for dinner.

334. ☐ Explain to your child how a traffic light works.
335. ☐ Teach your child the name of all the moving vehicles.
336. ☐ Make a calendar with your family pictures.
337. ☐ Teach how to tell the time.
338. ☐ Introduce your child to a collection.
339. ☐ Teach some proverbs and sayings.
340. ☐ Make a jigsaw puzzle with your kid.
341. ☐ Teach your child some knots.
342. ☐ Wash teeth with your child using your weak hand.
343. ☐ Build a coin tower.
344. ☐ Make a cake together.
345. ☐ Challenge your child to a run.
346. ☐ Pull a prank on your partner with your child.
347. ☐ Teach all the different musical instruments.

348. ☐ Write a letter to Santa Claus

349. ☐ Teach your child the names of all types of food.

350. ☐ *Californication*, by Red Hot Chili Peppers. Let your child listen to it.

Now, some space for you to fill...

351. ☐ _____

352. ☐ _____

353. ☐ _____

354. ☐ _____

355. ☐ _____

356. ☐ _____

357. ☐ _____

358. ☐ _____

359. ☐ _____

360. ☐ _____

361. ☐ _____

362. ☐ _____

363. ☐ _____

364. ☐ _____

365. ☐ _____

366. ☐ _____

367. ☐ _____

368. ☐ _____

369. ☐ _____

370. ☐ _____

371. ☐ _____

372. ☐ _____

373. ☐ _____

374. ☐ _____

375. ☐ _____

376. ☐ _____

377. ☐ _____

378. ☐ _____

379. ☐ _____

380. ☐ _____

381. ☐ _____

382. ☐ _____

383. ☐ _____

384. ☐ _____

385. ☐ _____

386. ☐ _____

387. ☐ _____

388. ☐ _____

389. ☐ _____

390. ☐ _____

391. ☐ _____

392. ☐ _____

393. ☐ _____

394. ☐ _____

395. ☐ _____

396. ☐ _____

397. ☐ _____

398. ☐ _____

399. ☐ _____

400. ☐ _____

Chapter Three

6 – 9 years old

Your child is now fully involved with other children at school so you may feel that you're somehow losing control on his/her development and growth. That is far from being true. You are still a crucial element in his/her psychological and social development. At this stage of your child's growth you should be playing and teaching a lot. You will see what a good teacher does at school to keep children entertained. If you will do so, your child will adore you. And maybe the next stage will be easier to face.

401. ☐ Calm your child about one of his/her fears.

402. ☐ Don't give him/her a smartphone.

403. ☐ Keep the 'goodnight kiss' tradition. Or establish it.

404. ☐ Keep the secret about Santa Claus.

405. ☐ Watch documentaries to learn animal behaviour.

406. ☐ Make some researches about the United States, Canada, Brazil, Mexico, Peru and Argentina.

407. ☐ Make some research about the United Kingdom, Ireland, Spain, France, Italy and Greece.

408. ☐ Make some research about Australia and New Zealand.

409. ☐ Make some research about India, Israel, Russia, China and Japan.

410. ☐ Make some research about South Africa, Nigeria, Kenya, Morocco and Egypt.

411. ☐ Teach your child some grammar.

412. ☐ Send your child to a summer camp.

413. ☐ Witness the fall of a milk tooth.

414. ☐ Bring your child to a concert.

415. ☐ *Clandestino*, by Manu Chao. Let your child listen to it.

416. ☐ Listen to Italian singers: Francesco De Gregori, Fabrizio De André, Vasco Rossi, Luciano Ligabue, Gino Paoli, Lucio Dalla, Francesco Guccini, Pierangelo Bertoli, Roberto Vecchioni, Giorgio Gaber, Fabio Concato, Lucio Battisti, Franco Battiato, Rino Gaetano, Jovanotti, Caparezza...

417. ☐ Show your child this book. Tell him/her that if you want to achieve something, it's better if you plan it before.

418. ☐ Educate your child to leave his/her seat on public transport to elderly people or pregnant women.

419. ☐ Explain your child the persuasive action of advertisement.

420. ☐ Educate your child to honesty.

421. ☐ Stimulate your child to play also with children of the opposite sex. Don't force him/her, just stimulate.

422. ☐ Tell your child the incredible story of Alex Zanardi.

423. ☐ Buy your child some stickers.

424. ☐ Prepare some sketches to entertain the relatives at family meetings.

425. ☐ Organize a surprise party to your partner with your child's help.

426. ☐ Let your child try the Scout movement.

427. ☐ Tell your child about his/her great grandparents.

428. ☐ Tell your child about the time when his/her mum was pregnant.

429. ☐ Give your child a diary to write thoughts and reflections.

430. ☐ Tell your child about your travels.

431. ☐ Tell your child about the time when you were his/her age.

432. ☐ Teach your child to count money so that they don't cheat him/her.

433. ☐ Teach him/her how to hang clothes properly.

434. ☐ Teach your child the names of the streets around your home.

435. ☐ Teach your child how to set the table for lunch and dinner.

436. ☐ Teach your child how to clean the bathroom.

437. ☐ Teach your child to read a clock. This time for real. Not just like in number 337.
438. ☐ Let your child help you in the storage room.
439. ☐ Teach your child the most important emergency numbers.
440. ☐ Fold the sheets with your child.
441. ☐ Teach your child to load and unload the dishwasher (if you are lucky enough to have one).
442. ☐ Let your child sweep the floor.
443. ☐ Let your child take an elevator alone.
444. ☐ Let your child go and buy some milk.
445. ☐ Let your child search for words on a paper dictionary.
446. ☐ Teach your child how to open wine and sparkling wine bottles.
447. ☐ Teach your child how to juggle some balls.

448. ☐ Teach your child some balance games.

449. ☐ Let your child start playing some instrument.

450. ☐ Teach your child to give easy instruction to a dog.

451. ☐ Teach your child to jump the rope.

452. ☐ Bring your child to the cinema.

453. ☐ *Hook*, by Steven Spielberg. Watch it with your child.

454. ☐ *The Family Man*, by Brett Ratner. Watch it with your child.

455. ☐ *Independence Day*, by Roland Emmerich. Watch it with your child.

456. ☐ Watch the *Harry Potter*'s saga.

457. ☐ Watch the *Star Wars* saga.

458. ☐ Watch *The Lord of the Rings* saga.

459. ☐ Watch all Robin Williams' movies.

460. ☐ Watch some Laurel and Hardy's sketch.

461. ☐ Make a cooking day with your family.

462. ☐ Bring your child to the thermal baths.

463. ☐ Fly a kite with your child.

464. ☐ Play some videogames together.

465. ☐ Play with the sunlight and with hand lens.

466. ☐ Play volleyball.

467. ☐ Play basketball.

468. ☐ Go to an observatory to watch the sky with a telescope.

469. ☐ Play with a frisbee.

470. ☐ Make a running race with your child.

471. ☐ Go to a beach with high waves.

472. ☐ Teach your child to stretch muscles.

473. ☐ Make a slide with a bobsled.

474. ☐ Let your child climb a rope.

475. ☐ Challenge your child to jog half a mile without stopping.

476. ☐ Bring your child to a waterfall.

477. ☐ Play chess with your child.

478. ☐ Teach your child some hand tricks.

479. ☐ Teach your child some card games.

480. ☐ Play 'Subbuteo' with your child.

481. ☐ Play 'Monopoly' with your child.

482. ☐ Play 'Clue' with your child.

483. ☐ Play 'Uno' with your child.

484. ☐ Play 'Guess who?' with your child.

485. ☐ Play 'Pictionary' with your child.

486. ☐ Play on a Tangram with your child.

487. ☐ Play Checkers.

488. ☐ Play 'hangman' with your child.

489. ☐ Teach and play 'Tic-Tac-Toe' with your child.

490. ☐ Teach and play the Battleship game.

491. ☐ Play the game of the Goose.
492. ☐ Play 'Connect Four' with your child.
493. ☐ Play Mikado with your child.
494. ☐ Don't talk during one day. Play with your child.
495. ☐ Invert your hands during one day. Play with your child.
496. ☐ Challenge your child to spit olive stones as far as possible.
497. ☐ Let your child give some of his/her toys to a charity organization.
498. ☐ Make a castle with cards.
499. ☐ Make a picnic with your child.
500. ☐ Make some pizza with your child.
501. ☐ Cook pasta with your child.
502. ☐ Make a Spanish Tortilla with your child.
503. ☐ Teach your child to make coffee.

504. ☐ Cook popcorn at home.

505. ☐ Teach yor child how to eat roasted sunflower seeds.

506. ☐ Let your child taste his/her first mate (infusion).

507. ☐ Enjoy some fireworks.

508. ☐ Bring your child to the stadium to watch football.

509. ☐ Bring your child to watch some athletics.

510. ☐ Bring your child to a car race.

511. ☐ Watch the Olympic Games.

512. ☐ Go to the park to pick up some trash.

513. ☐ Go to a restaurant to eat some traditional food.

514. ☐ Eat with sticks, just like the Japanese do.

515. ☐ Bring your child to a comedy show.

516. ☐ Show your child some rugby games (with experts, if needed).
517. ☐ Watch the New Zealand 'Haka' before a rugby match.
518. ☐ Listen to a classical music concert.
519. ☐ Let your child know the most famous national anthems.
520. ☐ Play repeat-spell-repeat.
521. ☐ Teach meditation and breathing control.
522. ☐ Study the times tables together.
523. ☐ Make a glass of salty water evaporate.
524. ☐ Make a circuit with a battery.
525. ☐ Explain density with some experiments with different liquids.
526. ☐ Teach your child to make easy Math calculation.

527. ☐ Teach your child the geography of your country.

528. ☐ *Raro*, by Cuarteto de Nos. Let your child listen to it.

529. ☐ Teach your child to make a press review.

530. ☐ Teach your child how to read a physical and political map.

531. ☐ Teach your child the flags of the different countries of the world.

532. ☐ Teach your child some History.

533. ☐ Teach your child how to read the Roman numerals.

534. ☐ Try to explain your child the Second World War and the Holocaust (*Shoah* in Hebrew).

535. ☐ Teach your child how to digit on a QWERTY keyboard.

536. ☐ Teach your child the theory of colours and how to mix them.
537. ☐ Teach your child how sexual reproduction works.
538. ☐ Teach the importance of good nutrition.
539. ☐ Teach your child about the Mexican painter Frida Khalo.
540. ☐ Bring your child to a Picasso's exhibition.
541. ☐ Bring your child to a contemporary art exhibition.
542. ☐ Establish a day in a month in which you only speak another language.
543. ☐ Explain your child how a State works and the separation of powers.
544. ☐ Make some research about different topics.
545. ☐ Watch a Sun eclipse.
546. ☐ Let your child prepare breakfast for you.

547. ☐ Invite some of your child's friends to come home and have lunch together.

548. ☐ Teach your child the Solar System.

549. ☐ Explain your child that some TV show use actors.

550. ☐ *Supernatural*, by Santana. Let your child listen to it.

Now, some space for you to fill...

551. ☐ _____

552. ☐ _____

553. ☐ _____

554. ☐ _____

555. ☐ _____

556. ☐ _____

557. ☐ _____

558. ☐ _____

559. ☐ _____

560. ☐ _____
561. ☐ _____
562. ☐ _____
563. ☐ _____
564. ☐ _____
565. ☐ _____
566. ☐ _____
567. ☐ _____
568. ☐ _____
569. ☐ _____
570. ☐ _____
571. ☐ _____
572. ☐ _____
573. ☐ _____
574. ☐ _____
575. ☐ _____
576. ☐ _____

577. ☐ _____
578. ☐ _____
579. ☐ _____
580. ☐ _____
581. ☐ _____
582. ☐ _____
583. ☐ _____
584. ☐ _____
585. ☐ _____
586. ☐ _____
587. ☐ _____
588. ☐ _____
589. ☐ _____
590. ☐ _____
591. ☐ _____
592. ☐ _____
593. ☐ _____

594. ☐ _____

595. ☐ _____

596. ☐ _____

597. ☐ _____

598. ☐ _____

599. ☐ _____

600. ☐ _____

Chapter Four

10 – 15 years old

Children at this stage are changing everything, from their physical body to the way they think and behave. It could be difficult to keep managing a positive and consistent relationship with them because they tend to be a bit elusive with adults. That's the tough beauty of adolescence! Anyway, never forget they are still young kids. Keep eyes open and stimulate their autonomy without losing control. Good luck and enjoy the ride. In this section of the list you will find many suggestions for movies, songs and topics of discussion. Try and do them with care. Don't be superficial. Apart from that, most of the work is done. And if things get bad, think that it's just a phase.

601. ☐ Get involved in one of his/her passions.

602. ☐ Let your child choose their clothes.

603. ☐ Give autonomy, but don't lose intimacy.

604. ☐ Help your child not to surrender to videogames addiction.

605. ☐ Buy your child a microscope.

606. ☐ Buy your child a drone.

607. ☐ Learn something you didn't know from your child.

608. ☐ Have fun with the incredible story of the Australian skater Steven Bradbury.

609. ☐ Try and explain your child what life is.

610. ☐ Try and answer his/her questions.

611. ☐ Test his/her ideas within a political compass.

612. ☐ Tell your child about the Buddhist Philosophy.

613. ☐ Tell your child about drug use.

614. ☐ Tell your child about religion.

615. ☐ Tell your child about gambling addiction.

616. ☐ Tell your child about smoking.

617. ☐ Tell your child about the risks of alcohol.

618. ☐ Tell your child about the risks of medical drugs.

619. ☐ Teach your child the difference between winter time and daylight-saving time.

620. ☐ Tell your child about the different time zones.

621. ☐ Teach your child how to read a nutrition facts on labels.

622. ☐ *School of Rock*, by Richard Linklater. Watch it with your child.

623. ☐ Go and play paintball with your child.

624. ☐ Write a song together.

625. ☐ Be sure your child is able to peel an apple.

626. ☐ Bring your child abroad.

627. ☐ Stimulate your child to find a summer or a weekend job.

628. ☐ Bring your child to the hairdresser/hairstylist.

629. ☐ Let your child sleep at one of his/her friend's house.

630. ☐ Stimulate your child to improve his/her handwriting.

631. ☐ Stimulate your child to save money for a specific purpose.

632. ☐ Write a letter together.

633. ☐ Bring your child to have a swim at night.

634. ☐ Organize a party in the park.

635. ☐ Stimulate your child to do something nice to a classmate or a friend.

636. ☐ Ask your child to write a poem.

637. ☐ Bring your child to a public library.

638. ☐ If your child is a girl, buy her a flower for her first menstruation.

639. ☐ Educate to tip and respect people's work.

640. ☐ Teach your child the importance of time and punctuality.

641. ☐ Teach your child the importance of money.

642. ☐ Teach your child the importance of keeping a promise.

643. ☐ Teach your child excellence, not perfection.

644. ☐ Teach respect for elderly people.

645. ☐ Teach respect for people who suffers.

646. ☐ Teach respect for people who made mistakes.

647. ☐ Teach your child some strategies to keep calm.

648. ☐ Teach your child to ration duty and pleasure.
649. ☐ Show your child the risks of speed.
650. ☐ Show your child the risks of two wheels vehicles.
651. ☐ Teach your child to be assertive and polite.
652. ☐ Teach your child to be quiet when there's no need to talk.
653. ☐ Teach your child to be confident, not overconfident.
654. ☐ Explain your child what you think about permanent tattoos.
655. ☐ Explain your child what you think about piercings.
656. ☐ Discuss about bullying and cyber-bullying.
657. ☐ Teach your child that not doing anything is being an accomplice.

658. ☐ Teach how to spot fake news.

659. ☐ Teach your child the Plato's Myth of the Cave.

660. ☐ Teach your child some body language.

661. ☐ Teach your child how to fire a small firecracker.

662. ☐ Let your child drive the car in an open, safe and empty space.

663. ☐ Teach your child to write an e-mail.

664. ☐ Teach your child to write in paragraphs.

665. ☐ Teach your child to light and control a fire.

666. ☐ Teach your child how to change strings in a guitar.

667. ☐ *Philadelphia*, by Jonathan Demme. Watch it with your child.

668. ☐ *The Good, the Bad and the Ugly*, by Sergio Leone. Watch it with your child.

669. ☐ *Life is Beautiful*, by Roberto Benigni. Watch it with your child.

670. ☐ *All About My Mother,* by Pedro Almodóvar. Watch it with your child.

671. ☐ Watch an action movie.

672. ☐ Watch some Woody Allen's movie with your child.

673. ☐ Watch some Steven Spielberg's movies with your child.

674. ☐ Watch some Stanley Kubrick's movies with your child.

675. ☐ Watch *the Matrix* saga.

676. ☐ Watch the *Indiana Jones* saga.

677. ☐ Watch the *Back to the Future* saga.

678. ☐ Watch *The Simpsons* with your child.

679. ☐ Bring your child to a street demonstration.

680. ☐ Climb a mountain with your child.

681. ☐ Bring your child to a Comics fair.

682. ☐ Make a big jigsaw puzzle with your child (at least 500 pieces).

683. ☐ *Apollo 13*, by Ron Howard. Watch it with your child.

684. ☐ *Matilda*, by Denny DeVito. Watch it with your child.

685. ☐ *Mary Poppins*, by Robert Stevenson. Watch it with your child.

686. ☐ *Bedknobs and Broomsticks*, by Robert Stevenson. Watch it with your child.

687. ☐ *The Mummy*, by Steven Sommers. Watch it with your child.

688. ☐ *The Truman Show*, by Peter Weir. Watch it with your child.

689. ☐ *Home Alone*, by Chris Columbus. Watch it with your child.

690. ☐ Ride a tandem bike together.

691. ☐ Make an apnoea challenge with your child.

692. ☐ Exercise together.

693. ☐ Make an herbal liquor together.

694. ☐ Make a painting together.

695. ☐ Make arm wrestling with your child.

696. ☐ Make a swimming challenge against your child.

697. ☐ Tell your child something personal about your adolescence.

698. ☐ Tell your child about the relationship you had with your parents when you were a kid.

699. ☐ Play 'Risk' with your child.

700. ☐ Play 'Taboo' with your child.

701. ☐ Go out for a dinner alone with your child and let him/her decide where to go.

702. ☐ Cook on a campfire together.

703. ☐ Go and take a stroll outside at night.

704. ☐ Let your child taste Fernet. Just few drops.

705. ☐ Let your child taste coffee.

706. ☐ Let your child learn how to make a Mate infusion.

707. ☐ Go to a cycling race to support.

708. ☐ Watch another edition of the Olympic Games.

709. ☐ Make a night trip on a train.

710. ☐ Sleep in a tent for a few nights.

711. ☐ Watch a political talk show with your child.

712. ☐ Let your child wash dishes for a week

713. ☐ Bring your child to a flea market.

714. ☐ Paint a t-shirt together.

715. ☐ Be sure your child is able to throw trash in the correct container.

716. ☐ Teach your child some minimalist game.

717. ☐ Let your child massage your back.

718. ☐ Let your child try some exotic fruit.

719. ☐ Teach your child to write a form.

720. ☐ A song your child should know by heart: *Sultans of Swing,* by Dire Straits.

721. ☐ A song your child should know by heart: *Father and Sons*, by Cat Stevens.

722. ☐ A song your child should know by heart*: Friday I'm in Love*, by The Cure.

723. ☐ A song your child should know by heart: *Wannabe*, by the Spice Girls

724. ☐ A song your child should know by heart: *Imagine*, by John Lennon

725. ☐ A song your child should know by heart: *Bohemian Rapsody*, by Queen.

726. ☐ A song your child should know by heart: *Don't look back in anger*, by Oasis.

727. ☐ A song your child should know by heart: *Wish you Were Here*, by Pink Floyd.

728. ☐ A song your child should know by heart: *Something*, by The Beatles.

729. ☐ A song your child should know by heart: *(I can't get no) Satisfaction*, by Rolling Stones.

730. ☐ A song your child should know by heart: *Your Song*, by Elton John.

731. ☐ A song your child should know by heart: *Angels*, by Robbie Williams.

732. ☐ A song your child should know by heart: *The Scientist*, by Coldplay.

733. ☐ A song your child should know by heart: *Stairway to Heaven*, by Led Zeppelin.

734. ☐ A song your child should know by heart: *Castle on the Hill*, by Ed Sheeran.

735. ☐ A song your child should know by heart: *God Save the Queen*, by Sex Pistols.

736. ☐ A song your child should know by heart: *Country Roads*, by John Denver.

737. ☐ A song your child should know by heart: *Have You Ever Seen the Rain?,* by the Creedence.

738. ☐ A song your child should know by heart: *The Passenger*, by Iggy Pop.

739. ☐ A song your child should know by heart: *Hotel California*, by the Eagles.

740. ☐ A song your child should know by heart: *Perfect Day*, by Lou Reed.

741. ☐ A song your child should know by heart: *Streets of Philadelphia*, by Bruce Springsteen

742. ☐ A song your child should know by heart: *Stand by me*, by Ben E. King.

743. ☐ A song your child should know by heart: *Come as You are*, by Nirvana.

744.   ☐ A song your child should know by heart:

Sweet Home Alabama, by Lynyrd Skynyrd.

745.   ☐ A song your child should know by heart:

Nothing else Matters, by the Metallica.

746.   ☐ A song your child should know by heart:

Imitation of Life, by R.E.M.

747.   ☐ A song your child should know by heart:

Blowin' in the Wind, by Bob Dylan.

748.   ☐ A song your child should know by heart:

Wonderful World, by Louis Armstrong

749.   ☐ A song your child should know by heart: Mrs

Robinson, by Simon and Garfunkel.

750.   ☐ A song your child should know by heart:

Where is the Love?, by the Black Eyed Peas.

Now, some space for you to fill...

751.   ☐ _____

752.   ☐ _____

753. ☐ _____

754. ☐ _____

755. ☐ _____

756. ☐ _____

757. ☐ _____

758. ☐ _____

759. ☐ _____

760. ☐ _____

761. ☐ _____

762. ☐ _____

763. ☐ _____

764. ☐ _____

765. ☐ _____

766. ☐ _____

767. ☐ _____

768. ☐ _____

769. ☐ _____

770. ☐ _____

771. ☐ _____

772. ☐ _____

773. ☐ _____

774. ☐ _____

775. ☐ _____

776. ☐ _____

777. ☐ _____

778. ☐ _____

779. ☐ _____

780. ☐ _____

781. ☐ _____

782. ☐ _____

783. ☐ _____

784. ☐ _____

785. ☐ _____

786. ☐ _____

787. ☐ _____

788. ☐ _____

789. ☐ _____

790. ☐ _____

791. ☐ _____

792. ☐ _____

793. ☐ _____

794. ☐ _____

795. ☐ _____

796. ☐ _____

797. ☐ _____

798. ☐ _____

799. ☐ _____

800. ☐ _____

Chapter Five

Things to do anywhere, anytime

This is possibly the most important chapter of the book. Here you will find the guidelines for the perfect parenting. If only I had ever accomplished just a 12% of all this, I would have been 'Father of the Year' for the last two decades. Take a look!

801. ☐ Provide your child with shelter.

802. ☐ Provide your child with therapy, if needed.

803. ☐ Love your child.

804. ☐ Be a good example.

805. ☐ Keep moments for yourself.

806. ☐ Ask for help or cooperation of other people.

807. ☐ Don't contradict your partner in front of your child. Discuss it later.

808. ☐ Don't deprive your child from his/her family members.

809. ☐ Learn as much as you can about everything.

810. ☐ Have fun together.

811. ☐ Make videos to show your child when he/she is grown up.

812. ☐ Be proud of your him/her.

813. ☐ Don't be afraid of correcting your child.

814. ☐ Don't be afraid of saying 'no'.

815. ☐ Don't be afraid, in general. Always convey enthusiasm and optimism.

816. ☐ Stop smoking and saying swear words.

817. ☐ Don't post pictures of your child online.

818. ☐ Don't overprotect him/her.

819. ☐ Don't treat your child as a divinity.

820. ☐ Be there when your child needs you.

821. ☐ Don't lose your cool with him/her.

822. ☐ Regret if you made a mistake towards him/her. But go on.

823. ☐ When your child is playing with some peers, don't interfere.

824. ☐ If they are doing something wrong or dangerous, stop them and call other parents.

825. ☐ Encourage your child to study.

826. ☐ Encourage efforts, not just results.

827. ☐ Keep talking with your child during his/her growth.

828. ☐ Answer his/her questions, but don't invent answers.

829. ☐ Stimulate your child to focus and fight for what he/she wants.

830. ☐ Buy him/her birthday presents.

831. ☐ Teach your child to respect animals.

832. ☐ Teach your child to respect others.

833. ☐ Teach your child to respect the environment.

834. ☐ Keep his/her secrets.

835. ☐ Teach your child to understand rules.

836. ☐ Stimulate your child's self-esteem.

837. ☐ Educate your child to respect your intimacy, your times, your needs.

838. ☐ Don't indulge all your child's whims.

839. ☐ Educate your child to enjoy the little things.

840. ☐ Let your child interact with others as much as possible.

841. ☐ Introduce your child to music.

842. ☐ Introduce your child to cinema.

843. ☐ Introduce your child to sport.

844. ☐ Introduce your child to art.

845. ☐ Be rational, if you want to educate your child to rationality.

846. ☐ Teach your child to be conscious with money.

847. ☐ Introduce your child to Emotional Intelligence.

848. ☐ Travel with your child as much as possible.

849. ☐ Set family traditions and stick to them.

850. ☐ Don't take life too seriously.

Chapter Six

Things to do around the world

Travelling around the world is a real privilege. Visiting new places, tasting new food and moving around the globe is probably the most intense way to increase experiences and get a deeper perspective on yourself and on reality.

I really hope you will be able to do at least some of these wonderful activities with your child.

851. ☐ Climb the Eiffel Tower in Paris, France.

852. ☐ Eat Sushi in Tokyo, Japan.

853. ☐ Spot a Geisha in Kyoto, Japan.

854. ☐ Visit the Niagara Falls.

855. ☐ Visit Cuba.

856. ☐ Make a Safari in the Serengeti-Park in Tanzania.

857. ☐ Visit the Gates of Hell in Turkmenistan.

858. ☐ Enjoy the coral reef in Mozambique.

859. ☐ Go to the Jazz Festival in New Orleans, US.

860. ☐ Make a thermal bath in Budapest, Hungary.

861. ☐ Visit the Old City in Jerusalem, Israel.

862. ☐ Take a picture with the Little Mermaid in Copenhagen, Denmark.

863. ☐ Eat a Kebab in Istanbul, Turkey.

864. ☐ Visit Galicia, Spain.

865. ☐ Take a picture to The White House, in Washington, US.

866. ☐ Visit Alaska.

867. ☐ Cross the Golden Gate Bridge in California, US.

868. ☐ Visit the Sequoia National Park, California, US.
869. ☐ Visit the Cliffs of Moher in Ireland.
870. ☐ Eat a Sacher-torte cake in Wien, Austria.
871. ☐ Visit the Guinness Museum in Dublin, Ireland.
872. ☐ Visit Nepal.
873. ☐ Climb the Empire State Building in New York City, US.
874. ☐ Place a bet in Las Vegas, US.
875. ☐ Visit South Africa.
876. ☐ Have a bicycle ride in Amsterdam, the Netherlands.
877. ☐ Explore Patagonia, Argentina.
878. ☐ Visit Corsica, France.
879. ☐ Go to the disco in Tel Aviv, Israel.
880. ☐ Go to San Siro Stadium in Milan, Italy.

881. ☐ Have a ride on a dromedary in the Sahara Desert.
882. ☐ Go shopping in the Marrakech Souk, Morocco.
883. ☐ Eat some Pasteis de Belem in Lisbon, Portugal.
884. ☐ Have a bath in the Dead Sea, Israel.
885. ☐ Drink a beer in Belgium.
886. ☐ Go to the Octoberfest in Munich, Germany.
887. ☐ Make a road trip in Australia.
888. ☐ Find a fado concert in Porto, Portugal.
889. ☐ Go to the Old Trafford Stadium in Manchester, England, UK.
890. ☐ See the Sufi Whirling Dervishes in Turkey.
891. ☐ Make a trekking in New Zealand.
892. ☐ Walk on the Chinese Wall.
893. ☐ Visit Hong Kong.

894. ☐ Visit South Korea.

895. ☐ Visit the ancient Inca city of Machu Picchu, Peru.

896. ☐ Visit San Petersburg, Russia.

897. ☐ Visit Plaza Mayor in Madrid, Spain.

898. ☐ Watch a Bull Race in Pamplona, Spain.

899. ☐ Visit Frida Khalo's Blue House in Mexico City, Mexico.

900. ☐ Visit Mongolia.

901. ☐ Watch a mountain stage of the Tour the France.

902. ☐ Eat *Empanadas* in the neighbourhood of La Boca in Buenos Aires, Argentina.

903. ☐ Visit the Santuario de las Lajas, Colombia.

904. ☐ Make a road trip along the Balkans.

905. ☐ Visit the Wasa Ship Museum in Stockholm, Sweden.

906. ☐ Visit the Easter Island, Chile.

907. ☐ Visit Tuscany, Italy.

908. ☐ Go to the Iguassu Falls, on the border between Argentina and Brazil.

909. ☐ Cross the Uyuni Salt Flat in Bolivia.

910. ☐ Get in the London Eye in London, England, UK.

911. ☐ Eat a pizza in Naples, Italy.

912. ☐ Visit the Beatles Museum in Liverpool, England, UK.

913. ☐ Take a funny picture beside the Leaning Tower of Pisa, Italy.

914. ☐ Eat oysters in Boston, US.

915. ☐ Visit Andalucía, Spain.

916. ☐ Go to Disneyland in Paris, France.

917. ☐ Watch an Ice Hockey match in Canada.

918. ☐ Go to a NBA match in the United States.

919. ☐ Visit Provence, France.

920. ☐ Visit Brittany, France

921. ☐ Get to North Cape, Norway.

922. ☐ Visit Greece.

923. ☐ Visit the Grand Canyon National Park in Arizona, US.

924. ☐ Drink some Tallisker Whiskey on the Isle of Skye, Scotland, UK.

925. ☐ See geysers and icebergs in Iceland.

926. ☐ Visit Vietnam.

927. ☐ Visit Laos.

928. ☐ Visit Cambodia.

929. ☐ Visit the Taj Mahal in India.

930. ☐ Visit Madagascar.

931. ☐ Meet Santa Claus in Lapland, Finland.

932. ☐ Visit the Red Square and the Kremlin in Moscow, Russia.

933. ☐ Visit the city of Petra, Jordan.

934. ☐ Visit Auschwitz, Poland.

935. ☐ Eat Ćevapi in Sarajevo, Bosnia and Herzegovina.

936. ☐ Visit Yemen.

937. ☐ Cross the Brandenburg Gate in Berlin, Germany.

938. ☐ Visit the banks of River Ganges in Varanasi, India.

939. ☐ Visit the Jewish Cemetery in Prague, Czech Republic.

940. ☐ Visit Bangkok, Thailand.

941. ☐ Visit Wieliczka Salt Mine, Poland.

942. ☐ Visit the Pyramids of Giza, Egypt.

943. ☐ Go to Rio de Janeiro, Brazil, on Carnival.

944. ☐ Taste mate in Uruguay.

945. ☐ Visit Venezuela.

946. ☐ Visit the Victoria Falls in Zambia.

947. ☐ Spot wild animals in Botswana.

948. ☐ Visit Sicily, Italy.

949. ☐ Sail to Antarctica from South America.

950. ☐ Visit Rome, Italy. Try to do all the things from the last chapter!

Chapter Seven

Things to do in Rome, Italy

Rome is a city that you won't ever forget. It's indescribably full of great activities to do. The suggestions that I put in this chapter are the 50 most interesting and unforgettable activities that anyone should do in Rome. Anyone, not just tourists.

It takes time to do everything so I recommend to spend at least 10 days in the city to be sure that you don't miss anything and you take your time to check all the items. Rome is really big and it's worth the few more days that you will spend visiting its attractions. I promise you won't regret.

In the unlikely hypothesis you wrongfully feel you've seen enough, there are a bunch of interesting places around Rome to be visited too. Just check them on the internet and keep having fun!

951. ☐ Visit San Peter's square and Basilica, climb its dome and visit the Vatican Museums. The Vatican State is not technically part of Rome, being an Independent State, but I don't care. Forgive me.

952. ☐ Eat your bag lunch under the Castel Sant'Angelo.

953. ☐ Watch the Capitoline wolf on the *Campidoglio*.

954. ☐ Enjoy the design of *Piazza del Campidoglio* and find the same design on the back of a 50 cents coin.

955. ☐ Visit the Capitoline Museums.

956. ☐ Put a hand in the Mouth of Truth (*Bocca della Verità*) and enter the *Santa Maria in Cosmedin* church to enjoy the Cosmati floor.

957. ☐ Take a stroll around the ruins of the Forum Holitorium.

958. ☐ Throw a coin in the Trevi Fountain. At night the fountain looks much better.

959. ☐ Climb to the Quirinal Palace (*Quirinale*), the official residence of the President of the Italian Republic.

960.   ☐ Dodge street vendors in Trinità dei Monti. Enjoy the beautiful 'Fountain of the Boat' (*Fontana della Barcaccia*).

961.   ☐ Climb the Janiculum (*Gianicolo*) from Trastevere and enjoy the panorama from in front of *Il Fontanone* ('the big fountain').

962.   ☐ Go to the Janiculum Hill to witness the cannon shot at 12 o'clock.

963.   ☐ Visit the Pantheon and have a *Granita di caffè con panna*.

964.   ☐ Have a dish of pasta in a Trastevere restaurant.

965.   ☐ Watch in the spy-hole of the Villa del Priorato di Malta on the Aventine Hill (*Aventino*).

966.   ☐ Take a stroll in the Orange Trees Garden (*Giardino degli Aranci*) on the Aventine Hill.

967. ☐ Visit the Jewish Museum and the Synagogue (*Tempio Maggiore*).

968. ☐ Eat a *Ginetto* with chocolate at 'Boccione', a traditional pastry shop in the Jewish Quarter.

969. ☐ See the Turtle Fountain (*Fontana delle Tartarughe*) in Piazza Mattei.

970. ☐ Cross the Tiber and take a stroll on the Tiberine Island.

971. ☐ Visit the Colosseum and the Roman Forum.

972. ☐ Visit *Piazza Navona* and enjoy the stunning *Fontana dei Quattro Fiumi*.

973. ☐ Visit the San Peter in Chains church (*San Pietro in Vincoli*) and enjoy the sculpture of Michelangelo's Moses.

974. ☐ Visit the Coppedè quarter.

975. ☐ Climb the stairs from Piazza del Popolo to the Pincian Hill and enjoy the panorama from the Villa Borghese Gardens.

976. ☐ Visit *Piazza Venezia* and the Altar of the Fatherland (*Altare della Patria*).

977. ☐ Enjoy the forced perspective gallery by Borromini at the Galleria Spada.

978. ☐ Learn about philosopher Giordano Bruno at *Campo de' Fiori*.

979. ☐ Visit the district of EUR.

980. ☐ Visit the Parliament at *Montecitorio*.

981. ☐ Visit the archaeological remains in the *Palazzo Valentini's* basement.

982. ☐ Find Caravaggio's paintings in *Santa Maria del Popolo*, *San Luigi de' Francesi* and *Sant'Agostino* churches.

983. ☐ Visit the Protestant Cemetery in Testaccio, near the Pyramid of Cestius.

984. ☐ Visit the smallest church in Rome: *Santa Madonna dell'Archetto*.

985. ☐ Shiver in fear in the Capuchin Crypt on Via Veneto.

986. ☐ Have an Ice-cream in the enchanting neighbourhood of *Garbatella*.

987. ☐ Go to the flea market of *Porta Portese* on Sunday morning.

988. ☐ Visit the Christian Catacombs.

989. ☐ Take a stroll inside the *Via Sannio* market and visit San John's Basilica.

990. ☐ Visit the Basilica of San Paul's Outside the Walls.

991. ☐ Take a stroll on the Appian Way.

992. ☐ Visit Tor Marancia and enjoy its street art.

993. ☐ Visit the Galleria Borghese and enjoy Bernini's sculptures.

994. ☐ Go to the *Stadio Olimpico* (Olympic Stadium) for a match of a local team (A.S.Roma or S.S.Lazio).

995. ☐ Take a stroll in the Tre Fontane Abbey. Try their Trappist Beer and their chocolate.

996. ☐ Visit the House of Little Owls (*Casina delle civette*) at Villa Torlonia.

997. ☐ Visit the Basilica of St. Mary of the Angels and the Martyrs on a sunny day and enjoy the effect of the meridian line.

998. ☐ Enjoy the flat dome at Sant'Ignazio church.

999. ☐ Enjoy the 'robotic' painting by Rubens at *Santa Maria in Vallicella* church.

1000. ☐ Have a walk in the Circus Maximus.

Conclusions

Well, now that you have finished this book you have got just one last item to check. Are you ready?

1,001 ☐ Recommend this book to a couple of friends and have the perfect life you have always dreamed.

Or

1,001 ☐ Don't recommend this book to anyone and be a miserable for the rest of your life.

Just kidding!

Anyway, I really hope you have enjoyed my book!

Thank you.

Federico Lanari

A Special Thanks to

Suzanne Thompson